I0434704

To Dream and Hope

To Dream and Hope

Danuta Ryduchowski

Writers Club Press
San Jose New York Lincoln Shanghai

To Dream and Hope

All Rights Reserved © 2001 by Danuta Ryduchowski

No part of this book may be reproduced or transmitted
in any form or by any means, graphic, electronic, or
mechanical, including photocopying, recording, taping,
or by any information storage retrieval system,
without the permission in writing from the publisher.

Writers Club Press
an imprint of iUniverse.com, Inc.

For information address:
iUniverse.com, Inc.
5220 S 16th, Ste. 200
Lincoln, NE 68512
www.iuniverse.com

ISBN: 0-595-18898-2

Printed in the United States of America

Gray Eyes

Sometimes
when I try to recall
a shadow of a smile in your gray eyes
so friendly and wise, eyes
that will never look at me like this again
a pain takes a sharp knife in its hand
and pierces me
just at the bottom of my eyes.
And tears flow
But they never show
Instead they flow
Somewhere into a strange place
Drip by drip they flow
into my heart.

CHAPTER I

THE BIRTHDAY PARTY IS OVER!

I will always remember this day. It was Saturday and I was very busy. I was preparing meals for my husband's birthday party.

He was celebrating his 47th birthday.

All our friends were already invited. I wanted to make a special meal for them.

In fact, I wanted to prepare several "special" meals—some traditional Polish meals, and some "new country" meals. There will be a meal prepared according to the "Chinese" and "Spanish" cuisine and for sure, a huge,

"American born" turkey, stuffed with special filling, will be roasted to decorate our table.

Though I was very busy, I also knew that I was a "lucky girl."

My mother was visiting me from Poland, and she was such a great cook!

At least, I will not have to worry about "Polish cuisine" meals. She would cook them.

I glanced at my watch. It was after 12p.m.—My husband should be back from visit to his dermatologist's office in Fort Lee, New Jersey, anytime from now.

"Thanks God, he is such a healthy and strong man,"— I realized. "There should be nothing serious with him this time—all he had it was just a slight itching of skin. It will disappear after he takes the medications prescribed to him by his dermatologist."

We came to the United States in October 1983. My husband had never had any health problems. He never took any sick leave. With a few exceptions, he didn't need to visit any doctors. Some time ago, I remember, he has complained about a small sore in his mouth. He made appointment with a famous dermatologist who had an expensive office located at a very prestigious location in Manhattan. This doctor has disregarded his main complaint, as meaningless. He recommended some kind of over-the counter ointment to treat it.

Instead, he examined my husband's prostate. He found that it was substantially enlarged, and he started the prostate treatment.

Can you imagine a dermatologist who was pretending to treat an enlarged prostate?

Very expensive biweekly visits were scheduled at this doctor's office (This doctor advertised himself in a very popular, New York area's published, Polish newspaper- it is how my husband found him.)

Some special and expensive medicines were prescribed to my husband. After taking them he began to feel really sick! Additionally, he also became very scared, suspecting that he probably had the prostate cancer—his prostate was enlarged!

In the meantime, the small sore in his mouth has disappeared completely!

I advised my husband—" Take a second opinion. Do not trust a single diagnosis made by a dermatologist only."

"Ask another doctor for a second opinion. See an urologist! The urology doctor is supposed to be an expert, and he should treat your enlarged prostate."

My husband saw an urologist who had much less expensive office that was located in New Jersey. On the basis of a thorough examination and two days of extensive testing in a hospital, the urologist did not find anything serious with my husband's prostate.

"The prostate of almost every man over forty years old is enlarged to a certain degree," my husband was advised. "Your prostate is not unusually enlarged, and no benign growths, or presence of any tumor or cancer was discovered during the tests."

"As a preventive measure, you should be examined on a yearly basis. Currently, you do not need any special treatment or medication to treat your prostrate."—My husband was advised.

He immediately canceled his visits with the famous dermatologist in Manhattan.

He stopped taking the medications prescribed to him that made him to feel sick.

The dermatologist was deeply disappointed, but we learned an important lesson—one should always ask for a second opinion! Never trust just one doctor!

With an exception for the above visits to the doctors, my husband was always healthy and strong like a "rock."

In fact, it was I, who was a "sick weakling." I have had my gall bladder removed recently, and a surgery on my left leg. I frequently was getting cold, flu, and sore throat attacks. I was a "walking plethora" of the most popular, seasonal diseases.

I was a "poor, overworked" woman who was trying to keep several jobs; a professional civil/ structural engineer; real estate salesperson; my own business developer, etc. In addition to housekeeping duties that included raising of two extremely energetic sons, cooking for my entire family, and other general household duties, not to mention a house cleaning.

"At least, not being of good health," I thought,—"I was very lucky to have such a strong and healthy husband!"

"He always will be here to listen to my complaints about my health problems.

He will take care of me and take me to the doctor, when it is needed. At least, a one person in the family has to be strong and healthy. And, it will be him!"

For sure, during these ten years since our immigration to the United States, we had many other difficult and of a different nature than health, problems.

We didn't realize how tough it would be to start and survive during this beginning period of our immigration. My husband, who was a professional mechanical engineer, has gone through several unemployment periods during this time. I was luckier; being a professional civil/structural engineer. I always had more stable employment. Since beginning of my work in USA, it was I, who was changing jobs.

Last time, when my husband has lost his job, I had been employed, as a senior structural engineer, by a very reputable consulting engineering company. However, it was also a time when this consultant had a "slow—down time" -they were expecting some new engineering contracts to come.

Frankly speaking, I was not very busy, practically, there was almost no work for me to do—and with unemployed husband, a house mortgage to pay, payments for our older son's Michael private school, and our "baby" son Raymond's child care expenses, I was really nervous about this entire situation. At a first possible occasion, I accepted an offer from a BI- State public service Company that practically has never laid off any workers, in the eighty years' time. I hoped that we would be finally safe! What a mistake!

"This job would be more secure and provide a stable income and health benefits to my family,"—I hoped.

Additionally, I was planning to make a significant professional contribution to this public service company. I was really optimistic about my entire professional future, and I did not even want to dream about going into any other profession, including health guide writing.

In the meantime, my husband was going through a very hard time.

Very hard working, honest, and talented, he was needed and appreciated by his employers, when there was a lot of work to do. However, with his heavy foreign accent, honest and open "Slavic" heart, and his relatively short "American professional experience," he was either the first let "to go," when there was no work, or to become a "scape-goat" when one was needed.

Also, he recently went through a very stressful personal situation.

Both his parents have passed away, within six months time of each other. It was a real shock to him.

But he always smiled patiently, when I complained about my work environment, lack of professional satisfaction and recognition. He listened patiently, when I complained about his inability to keep a steady job. What a jerk I was!

When I was so easy to complain and cry, he never did the same. He always was quiet, friendly and supportive to me and to other people around him.

He was to reassure me, and support, when I was disappointed and sometimes having absolutely "enough of everything."

With a lot of stress that he was experiencing himself, he has never complained or had shown how difficult was his own life.

"But the bad times were finally over,"—I thought, while preparing meals for my husband's birthday party.

Life was so good for both of us, finally. Now, we both had relatively well paying and prestigious jobs. We both were registered professional engineers. With our hard work, we have achieved a "middle class" status. We had two cars, a house (with a large mortgage to pay), and our older son, Michael, was an honor student, constantly on a "Dean's List," at his college. Our "baby" son Raymond attended a kindergarten, and, though he was famous for his "misbehavior", for sure he would join his older brother on a Dean's List, in the future.

Things were going so well recently, that we had been able to afford a one-week vacation in Cancun, Mexico. We were postponing this event several times, but finally we went there. We had a lot of fun, swimming and snorkeling in the ocean. It was almost five weeks since we came back from this vacation, but we still had some tan from staying at the sunny Mexican beaches.

"Life is good,"—I thought.

"We deserve what we have, thanks to our talents, ambition, and hard work, and there is a birthday party today. Our friends are coming, and there will be a lot of joy, talk, and maybe even some dancing (Though my husband would not dance because he still had a "grieving time," after his parents' loss.)"

I had a glance at my watch again.

It was 1 p.m.- he was going to be late for lunch!

What was the reason?

"Maybe he had to wait at the doctor's office,"—I realized.—"Or some other problems kept him late." But, here he was, finally! Just on time for lunch—we would have it together.

While we sat down at the kitchen table, we all have listened to my husband's relation.

The doctor he saw, the New Jersey dermatologist, had examined his skin thoroughly (My husband's main complaint was his skin itching.) The doctor suspected that this itching was probably caused by a fungus infection (Recently, my husband had traveled intensively, on his company's business.) He suspected that though he was staying at very good hotels, he could possibly become infected there, maybe from some dirty towels?

The dermatologist took his skin's sample, and it would be tested in a medical laboratory.

"The doctor,"—my husband advised,—"Had asked me a very bizarre question. He asked if I were ever exposed to the hepatitis virus."

"I advised him,"—my husband continued his story,—"that I did not have any knowledge about being ever infected with hepatitis in the past. The doctor smiled, and asked me if my skin was always so yellowish."

The doctor advised my husband that the skin tests would be ready in about two weeks' time. Meanwhile, he prescribed to my husband some pills to swallow, and a skin ointment to apply on his skin. These medications should alleviate his skin itching. The doctor would contact my husband after the tests' results are ready, and the next office visit was preliminary scheduled. After the visit, my husband went to a drug store to buy prescribed to him medications. He had to wait for them at the local pharmacy. It was main reason why he was so late for lunch. He would start taking these medications immediately after the lunch.

We listened to his relation, while eating our meal.

I already knew that there should be nothing serious with his health. The doctor was an expert. He has examined my husband. The skin itching would disappear, after my husband takes all these special medicines.

Let's go with the party!

Our friends would be here soon!

However, my mother had a long look at my husband. After a while, she made her diagnosis; "Casimir, your eyes' whites are so yellow!"

"In my opinion, you do not have a skin infection. You have hepatitis!"

"You should see a "regular" family doctor immediately!"

"Casimir, the hepatitis is a very contagious disease, and it shouldn't be ignored!"

I again had a look at my husband. I have recently had some "thoughts" that his eyes' whites were more yellow than usually.

However, I remembered that when my brother Henry had hepatitis a long time ago, not only his skin and his eyes' whites were yellow. Also, the skin under his fingernails was very yellow. It was not such a case with my husband. Also, my brother didn't complain about any skin itching (He was six years old, when he was diagnosed with the hepatitis.) And skin itching was my husband's main complaint!

Anyhow, maybe, my mother was right; his eyes' whites were really yellowish!

It would be better if he sees a "regular" doctor, as soon as possible!

However, it was a Saturday. Our family doctor's office was closed on Saturdays. In addition, our doctor just went on a vacation, and he wouldn't be back within a two weeks' time. "What should we do?" Then, I realized that there was an "emergency" medical office in our town. It was open on Saturdays and Sundays. They were good doctors, too. I often visited this place when my "baby" son Raymond had a sudden attack of fever or a whopping cough. The emergency doctors have already helped us several times in the past. My husband should see them immediately.

When my husband went to see an emergency doctor, I had, instead to continue cooking,

quick look into the medical encyclopedia. I was looking for a description of hepatitis.

"Here we are!"

The hepatitis symptoms include yellowishness of skin, eyes' whites, and skin itching!

"Skin itching,"—I realized—"My husband's main complaint was skin itching. So, he possibly is infected with hepatitis!"

Suddenly, I realized what was the cause of his infection. We just came back from a vacation in Mexico! We went to restaurants there!

"The poor fool,"—I thought,—"has eaten a special fish (As far as I remember, it was, probably, a sandfish.) I didn't eat this fish—he did. He has gotten a hepatitis virus. I have not got it!"

"Here we are"—this fish is also described in another encyclopedia. "If improperly cooked,"—the encyclopedia said,—"This fish (which often is infected with hepatitis virus), can cause hepatitis in humans!"

"In fact, a consumption of this fish already caused hepatitis in my husband! "—I realized.

My mother was right!

Meanwhile, over three hours have passed, and it was already after 4 p.m. The guests were supposed to arrive by 7 p.m.

"What should we do next?"—My husband just came back from an emergency medical office. The doctor has examined him. The doctor asked if my husband were a homosexual! According to this doctor, the gay men are more often exposed and have a better chance to become infected with a hepatitis and AIDS, due to their contacts with strangers and infected needles.

My husband was referred for further tests to the nearby hospital. His blood sample was taken, and the X- rays were made at the hospital.

Though it was too early to make final diagnosis, before the tests' results are available, the emergency doctor's preliminary diagnosis was almost done.

My husband was sick. Probably, he had a very serious disease called hepatitis, but the doctor was not able to advise, until the tests' results are available, what type of the hepatitis it was.

After visiting an emergency office, my husband went back home. The doctor advised him that he would contact him on Monday, after the hospital tests' results are available.

To me, one thing was sure!

There would be no 47th birthday party for my husband today!

I called all our friends. I told them that my husband had seen two doctors and was examined at the hospital.

"The symptoms were typical for a hepatitis, and though we were not sure, he probably had gotten this contagious disease,"—I advised our friends.

Everybody was invited and welcome, on his or her own risk, for the party (The gifts were already bought, and my mother and I, we were finally done with the cooking.)

Would anybody, please, come?

Nobody has volunteered—the birthday party was over!

CHAPTER II

THE DIAGNOSIS

Now, we had to wait till Monday for a diagnosis.

Believe me, for us it was a long, as a matter of fact, a very long weekend.

We tried to become organized—we all knew that hepatitis was a serious and contagious disease. But the doctor didn't advise us what we should do next. Should we, or shouldn't we go to work as usual (When my brother was sick, I was not allowed to attend school for a several weeks' time, as a preventive measure.)

However, it is America!

Nobody would pay you, if you were not working, and my sick leave didn't cover such unusual situation

I was facing now (I was paid a sick time, only when I was sick.) My husband had no paid sick leave. Our older son had to attend college classes, and since I had to work, our "baby" son Raymond should go to a kindergarten.

What should we do?

Let's wait till Monday!

Meanwhile, we decided that my husband should not take any medication prescribed to him by the dermatologist, until final diagnosis of his condition is made. Improper medication may additionally damage his liver, that was already attacked (as we suspected), by a hepatitis virus.

When Monday came finally, we all went on our daily chores. Even my husband, since the doctor hasn't forbidden him, decided to go to work (As usual, he had an urgent project to finish.)

It was almost a lunch time, when he called me— "Dana, the emergency doctor just called. Now, it appears that his diagnosis was more serious than the first one—I will have to be operated. Not only the hepatitis antibodies were found in my blood, but also, the bile duct's obstruction, probably a stone, was discovered by the x—ray tests."

He continued—"This obstruction was blocking a flow of bile from my gall bladder. The doctor advised that I should undergo an emergency operation, the gall bladder's removal, as soon as possible, at the local hospital. The doctor advised me that the time was of an essence—I must give him an answer today!"

"Wait, wait!"—I tried to calm him down.

"Let's become organized. You should tell your doctor that you would need more time and you cannot answer him today. Please advise him that you would call him very soon."

My husbands hang a receiver. I felt a surge of a weakness and panic, overwhelming me. The reason for this panic was not the presence of the hepatitis antibodies in my husband's blood. Also, a prospect of his emergency operation, a gall bladder's removal, didn't frighten me.

"An obstruction in the gall bladder or bile duct never belonged to the "terminal" diseases,"—I thought— "The operation should be an easy one."

The real reason for my panic was that this operation would be performed at the local hospital. We have already had a "special" experience with this hospital. My husband's aunt, invited by us on a tourist visa from Poland, had fallen on the ice in our driveway. She broke her knee. An emergency ambulance took her to this local hospital. After two days of her stay at this hospital, totally exhausted, she begged us to take her back home.

She stayed in one room with three other ladies. Two of them were in a pain and constantly crying. Our aunt couldn't sleep all these nights.

Additionally, she couldn't get a proper attention when needed because her English was very poor—she was in pain and couldn't get painkillers after she asked for them, etc.

Soon after she left the hospital, the bill arrived—the hospital charged us for a two weeks' of her stay— though she stayed there only three days.

We believed that we should only be charged for a "real" time of her stay. In response, we were advised that the hospital had a legal right to charge each patient "per case," and in her "case", she was "required" to stay in the hospital for a two weeks' time!

I did not want my husband to be operated in this hospital. Also, after our experience with the famous dermatologist who had such a prestigious office in Manhattan, I believed that my husband needed a "second opinion" of another doctor, before undergoing any major treatment or operation.

But what should we do?—Our family doctor was still on vacation!

Then, I have gotten a sudden idea! I had my gall-bladder removed at another hospital. I was staying, alone, in a clean, single room, and I got plenty of rest after my operation. Also, I believed that the surgeon, who performed my operation, was a real expert. I hadn't gotten any infection, and there were no problems or complications with my health after my operation. I called my doctor—unfortunately, he was sick. He was no longer admitting any new patients. Instead, he referred us to another surgeon.

My husband decided to get a second opinion from this surgeon.

He decided to advise the emergency doctor about his decision.

I do not remember the exact reason, but he has never had a chance to see this second surgeon. Probably, the doctor was too busy with other patients and operations, and my husband's visits were postponed several times. He couldn't wait any longer—he decided to visit a doctor, who was substituting our absent family doctor.

Doctor L., a young doctor, who has recently opened his practice in our township, had recognized, after reviewing my husband's x-ray tests' results that a more thorough examination would be needed, before a gall-bladder's removal operation is performed.

He referred my husband to doctor R., an expert in internal medicine, the gastroenterologist. My husband again underwent a number of new hospital tests, at this time, at the St. Mary Hospital in Passaic. He had to stay at this hospital twice; first for the CAT scan and x -ray tests, and then for an internal sounder probe (Diagnostic ERCP test.) The CAT Scan test didn't indicate on any growths in his abdominal area. The x—ray test indicated an obstruction in his bile duct. The internal sounder probe, ERCP test, indicated on a possible presence of cancer—the probability of carcinoma of the biliary tract (primary) was diagnosed.

An artificial tube/stent was temporarily inserted in my husband's bile duct. The insertion of this tube brought him an immediate relief—now, the bile could flow freely. The jaundice has disappeared immediately. My husband was feeling well again.

I was puzzled. I was very puzzled indeed!

"He saw so many doctors,"—I thought—" The dermatologist, the emergency doctor, the gastroenterologist."

All these doctors have investigated my husband. Each doctor gave him a different opinion. The first doctor has diagnosed him with a possible skin infection.

The second doctor advised that an emergency gall bladder's removal operation would be required due to the possibility of a stone presence in his bile duct.

The third doctor diagnosed cancer—the carcinoma of the biliary duct (primary) condition was suspected.

Which doctor was right?

What was the real problem with my husband?

CHAPTER III

CASIMIR GOES TO HOSPITAL

I didn't want to admit that my husband possibly might have cancer. To me, a diagnosis of cancer's presence sounded like a death sentence. In addition, on a basis of the tests already performed, no final diagnosis of the disease was made as yet. I believed that none of the doctors really knew what was going on with my husband!

Since they didn't know, there had to be nothing really serious with my husband's health—I tried to convince the two of us.

Meanwhile, our family doctor came back from a vacation. We were able to see him, finally. In fact, he wanted to see the two of us. He looked very worried, during this consultation. The diagnosis, he advised, though was not certain yet, was a very serious one. He reviewed the medical tests' results. A possibility of cancer, a pancreatic cancer, in addition to the biliary duct's cancer, couldn't be excluded. In his opinion, the artificial tube inserted in my husband's bile duct would adequately serve its purpose, if my husband were over 90 years old.

But, if my husband wanted to live, he would have to undergo an operation, as soon as

possible. Only after his abdomen is open, a real diagnosis of my husband's health problem could be made, we were advised.

The doctor gave my husband two options; he gave him a choice of two surgeons and hospitals.

The first choice was the Passaic General Hospital— our doctor was admitted for a practice in this hospital. He knew a very talented, innovative young surgeon, who was an operating surgeon at this hospital. This surgeon could operate on my husband. In addition, our family doctor would be able to participate in this operation, and later on, he would follow on my husband's recovery.

The second choice, we were advised, was doctor F.,—a surgeon operating at the Saint Barnabas Hospital in Livingston, New Jersey. Doctor F., according to our family doctor opinion, was a very experienced and talented surgeon. He enjoyed very good opinion among his patients.

The final choice decision belonged to my husband.

I didn't want to make any suggestions, to bring any ideas to him at this time.

I would never forgive myself, if an improper choice were made.

I waited for my husband's decision.

Finally, he advised that he wanted to make an appointment with Doctor F. He preferred to deal with a more experienced surgeon than with an innovative young one. He wanted to be operated at the Saint Barnabas hospital. He didn't want to postpone his operation any longer. He was ready for it and he wanted it to be done as soon as possible.

He made an appointment and saw doctor F.

After this visit, he looked very uneasy.

He looked, as if he were hiding something from me.

Later on, he advised that according to doctor F., a definite, real diagnosis of his health problem could be made only during the operation, after his abdomen was open.

If the obstruction in the bile duct were caused by a gallstone/ gall sand presence (we had hoped that it would be the case), the operation would be a very simple one. It shouldn't last more than two to three hours.

However, if the cancer, and specially, the pancreatic cancer were found, the operation would involve a removal of a portion of the pancreas, about half of the stomach, a removal of the portions of the surrounding intestines and, if needed, other organs. This would be a very serious operation, my husband was advised, and about 25% of the patients either do not survive it, or die soon after it. Also, this operation would take a much longer time than the gallbladder's removal.

According to doctor F., this operation would extent my husband's life, possibly up to two additional years. My husband sounded very serious, while giving me this relation. I tried to smile to him—for sure, it couldn't be, and there would be no cancer found. After all, the three doctors couldn't give us a definite diagnosis.

Was my husband having a cancer?—Malignant cancer of the pancreas?

No!—It was impossible!

Even if it were a pancreatic cancer, probably it was not the "worst," the most malignant type of cancer—maybe, it was just a benign cancer, one that wouldn't spread quickly?

I tried to interview my mother. She, with her old age experience (though she didn't have any medical education), was so knowledgeable in the medical field (She worked at one of the pediatric hospitals in Warsaw, as a medical clerk, for many years.)

During one of our occasional conversations, I mentioned to her that Casimir would have to go to the hospital for an operation.

"Casimir, why would he have to be operated?"— She asked. He only has hepatitis; there was never any need for an operation when one had hepatitis. Unless there was a serious damage to the liver, and it had to be replaced, nobody was ever operated for hepatitis!

"Mom,"—I told her—"Casimir either has gotten a gallstone obstructing his bile duct, or a cancerous growth, possibly even a pancreatic cancer."

First, she didn't understand this statement.

Then, she looked at me with the unbelieving eyes.

"He couldn't have gotten a cancer, not a cancer of the pancreas,"—she advised feebly.

"The pancreatic cancer is the worst possible cancer, a human being might get!

If he really has gotten a pancreatic cancer, he would be gone in a six months' time!"

"I didn't know anybody, who lived longer,"—she advised,—"after he or she was diagnosed and operated for the pancreatic cancer."

Now, it was my time to be shocked.

Now, I looked at her with the unbelieving eyes, and then suddenly, I realized -"She was right! She was probably right!"

My eyes were getting wetter, and wetter, and I had to run away from her bedroom.

I wanted to be alone. I needed to be alone.

I cried alone, in my bedroom. I told to myself—" This was not true! It was just a wrong diagnosis!"

"It couldn't be true! My husband couldn't have gotten this kind of cancer. The doctors have made a mistake, as usually, and it would be found out soon that they all were totally wrong!"

After calming myself down, I walked back to my mother's bedroom.

She was sitting on her bed, like an old, lifeless toy.

Only her arms were shaking, and large tears were flowing down her wrinkled cheeks.

After she saw me, she cried loudly;—"How stupid, how stupid of me it was!—I should have never told you these stupid things, Danusia!"

"I should have watched my mouth!"—she cried.

"Why did I tell you such a cruel thing!"

"My child!"

"I feel so sorry!"

"Mom,"—I told her, trying to calm her down.

"Casimir does not have the pancreatic cancer. It can not be the pancreatic cancer. The doctors do not know it yet, for sure, and they have just speculated that it could be a case. That it might be the case!"

"Mom,"-I told her- "I am sure that it will be found out, that it will turn out, that he only has gotten a gall-stone obstructing his bile duct."

I finally was able to convince both her and myself, that there was nothing serious with my husband—the operation would turn out a small gallstone, and this entire mess would be over soon! He will be fine in no time at all!

I also have tried to convince my husband that since a CAT Scan test hadn't shown any tumors, it would be only a gallstone, obstructing his bile duct.

But deeply inside, I felt a panic. I was scared, but I didn't want to admit it to anybody, even to myself, how worried I was. I tried to play it easy.

In the meantime, my husband was ready for an operation—he had to wait some time for the operating room and bed availability at the Saint Barnabas hospital.

Finally, we received an urgent call, on Saturday, March 27, from the hospital staff. The operating room would be available on Monday, March 29. My husband would have to report to the hospital on Sunday, by 3 p.m.

He was very calm and optimistic, as usual, after hearing that news.

On Saturday, he invited his brother and sister-in-law, who just came from Poland to visit their daughter in Detroit, and were staying with us for a couple of days, for a sight-seeing of Manhattan. He had shown them the Statue of Liberty. He spent most of the Saturday, trying to entertain them.

On Sunday, our son Michael, my brother-in-law Felix and I, escorted him to the hospital. I saw his surgeon, doctor F., for the first time (from a distance), but I was too nervous to talk to him. I tried my best to stay calm and to smile, thus assuring my husband, that after this stupid gallstone is removed and he gets better, we again would travel to Mexico for another wonderful vacation.

Finally, I waived him good bye, and had a last look at him when he was entering the hospital elevator. He smiled to me. I tried to smile to back to him but it was too much for me. No, he couldn't see me crying!

I turned back.

I couldn't stand it any longer. I couldn't resist a flow of sadness, and a despair that was overwhelming. I started to cry on my way to car.

I was free to cry now! He couldn't see it. I didn't want to show him, how upset I was!

I was afraid that my sadness would adversely affect him.

That it would make him more ill and weak.

Next day, it was the day of the operation. I tried to pretend that nothing really serious was happening to us on this day, but deeply inside I was a nervous wreck.

"After all, it was only a gallstone removal operation," —I tried to convince myself.

I already went through this experience myself—it was a very painful operation, but I was feeling well in a few weeks' time. Again, it would be nothing really serious with my husband. It has to be nothing serious with my husband today. He would be well in no time at all! He must be well—after all, he is so strong!

More important, this operation would confirm that he has never had any stupid pancreatic cancer! Finally, after four hours of waiting and counseling myself, I called the hospital.

I asked the hospital volunteer how was my husband doing.

I was convinced that his operation should be over, by this time, if it was just a simple gallstone's removal operation.

But my husband was still in the operation room, according to the volunteer's advice. However, I was told that everything was fine and under control—the volunteer would call me after the operation is over. There was nothing to be worried about!

However, I became very nervous. I couldn't wait patiently—calling the hospital every half an hour. Now, the line was busy most of the time. I had to wait on line. I couldn't get any information at all!

Finally, I couldn't take it any longer—I decided to rush to the hospital.

Soon after I arrived there, I was advised that the operation was almost nearing its end.

By 4 p.m., it was finally over—I was told that my husband had been transferred to the recovery room.

He was doing fine, I was advised.

I told to myself—this operation lasted too long!

It had to be something more serious than just the gallstone removal operation.

Anyhow, the good news was that my husband survived this operation.

The worst was over—everything would be well now!

I have waited, I do not remember for how long exactly, but probably for additional two hours. Then, the hospital staff escorted me to the intensive care unit where I could see my husband. I rushed to his room—and there he was!

He was very pale, but, otherwise, he looked perfectly normal, almost as if he had never had any operation. Sure, he had all these tubes, and other intravenous feeders, etc., connected to him. He resembled a large apparatus himself.

But he looked very energetic and animated (I learned later, that immediately after the operation, he was administered drugs and he was "high" on a morphine for several days.)

He laughed a lot, and joked, as he reported to me his awakening after the operation. Almost immediately after he woke up, he was requested to rise to a sitting position. He felt a terrible pang of pain, and immediately after it, he was given, intravenously, painkiller. Now, he felt no pain at all. He felt great!

Suddenly, he became very serious.

His face expression changed and he mentioned, trying to smile negligently,—"Danusia,

after I woke up, it was already after 4 p.m."

"This operation started very early in the morning. It was not just a simple gallstone removal operation, Danusia. This had to be much more serious operation!

I am sure that I was operated for pancreatic cancer!

I am positively sure, that the pancreatic cancer was found, after my abdomen was opened. It was the pancreatic cancer's tumor that was removed during this operation!"

CHAPTER IV

ONE NIGHT'S FLIGHT

After seeing my husband after the operation, and staying at his bedside till evening, I went back home. It was Monday evening.

Though slightly nervous, I generally felt a radiant jubilance. I felt happy!

Casimir was alive, though connected to all these tubes and pumps. He survived the operation! He didn't die during it.

He was doing better than 25% of the patients, dying during this operation. The worst was over! The future would be bright!

He would live a long life!

I called doctor F. on Tuesday morning, and talked to him about my husband's operation. The operation was successful, the doctor has advised. The cancerous growth was removed from my husband's pancreas. He was recovering fine.

I kept visiting my husband at the hospital every evening, and every day he looked better and stronger. On Thursday evening, on a third evening after his operation, he looked almost as if he had never had any operation.

This evening he advised me and our friends who were visiting him, that the artificial feeding tube and the artificial bladder duct would be disconnected from him. According to his doctors, he no longer needed these devices.

Also, on this Thursday afternoon, he was taken out from the painkiller, morphine.

This was great news! His progress was really encouraging!

With an exception for a slight irritation in his throat, caused by the displaced feeding tube, he looked perfect, when I kissed him a good bye.

This evening, I went back home totally relaxed. I felt completely satisfied with all the developments—my husband was operated, and his operation was successful!

The cancerous growth was removed from his pancreas and he was recovering fine, and he would be at home in no time of all!

Already, he looked so healthy!

Everything was under control!

He was in good hands and totally safe at his hospital.

Now, it was my turn to sleep well and relax, comforted by his satisfactory recovery.

However, I remember, that on this Thursday night I had a very bizarre sleeping dream.

In this dream, I saw a big screen. I was in a movie theater.

On this screen, I saw a beautiful, young, unknown to me lady.

She had a fair hair, and her face features were classically regular. She was a real beauty!

She saw me and she smiled and started to talk to me.

Frankly speaking, I didn't remember exactly what did she tell me.

But I remember that, suddenly, I also landed on this screen.

The movie, which I had been watching up to now, this movie, became a real life story—I was an actively participant in its action.

I was no longer an observer—I became an actor, myself. No, it was no longer a play—it was a story that was really happening to me.

I remember that I was trying to escape from somebody, who was chasing me.

It was a desperate flight. I was not alone—I kept a boy's hand in my hand. We were both running from an attacker. I did not remember who was this boy— was it my "baby" son Raymond or somebody else?

Then I realized suddenly—the chaser, the attacker, was not after me!

He was trying to grab the boy from me!

Already, the chaser was very close—he would steal the boy from me. He would separate us, forever!

Suddenly, I saw a possibility for an escape—I saw a house in front of me. I opened its

door and we run into this house.

We run into a long and a very dark corridor.

But the attacker was just behind us; he was getting closer to us! I had to run, quickly!

Suddenly, I saw a light at the end of the corridor. I immediately run into its direction. Then, I realized that this light was coming from a backyard that was behind the house.

My mother-in-law, who passed away more than a year ago, was standing in the backyard. I saw her—she was very, very real. She smiled to me. She would help me! She must help me! "Grandma! Grandma!"—I cried (From the moment our children were born, her official name became "Grandma"),—"Please help us!"

Please, free us from this attacker! Try to mislead him!

Please, tell him that we were not here!

Tell him that we have already run away from this house and we are on the street!

I turned back, and I run into the stairway, upstairs from the dark corridor. I started to climb the stairs.

But what was happening to me? I felt a sudden change!

Suddenly, there was no fear in me any longer!

I felt, that I was ready to fight!

I told to myself—"You stupid bastard! I will show you how to run away!"

"Why is it me who is running away from you? I will show you how to run! It should be you, running away from me, instead of me, running away from you!"

I wanted to fight! I was ready for a fight!

I turned back, and I attacked and run after the chaser.

There was no fear in me now! I felt the force that was making me strong! I felt that I was very strong, indeed!

This time, it was the attacker, the chaser, who was running away. He became scared! He turned back and run into the street. He wanted to disappear. He was trying to start his car!

He was driving away! I could not reach him!

I saw the hopelessness of this situation. There was no sense in chasing him any longer.

I told myself—let's write down his car license plates. Write down all the information you can get about him. Write down how he looks alike! Identify the bandit! Everybody should know him! And, in my sleeping dream, I started to write everything down. Then, my dream has changed, suddenly.

I was back in the Movie Theater. I was sitting in a chair and watching the screen.

The beautiful lady was on the screen again. She was very friendly and she smiled to me. I felt warmth, friendliness, and love radiating from her beautiful face. She was like a good angel. But what was happening to her?

I couldn't believe my eyes! Her face got numerous wrinkles, she was getting old! She was undergoing transformation so suddenly and quickly!

In fact, she started to crush down, to dissipate into minute pieces!

She was disappearing just before my eyes!— Suddenly, she was gone!

The screen in the Movie Theater was empty. The movie was over. I was in the Movie Theater alone. I was sitting in a chair; nobody was there.

I felt sadness and loneliness.

I felt an anxiety. I remember, I started to cry, shriek!

I cried—"Oh, no! You are dead! You are dead, and you came to me! You came to me

from another world! I saw dead people!"

Suddenly, I was awoke, still screaming and yelling.

I felt tears flowing down my cheeks. My cheeks were wet. My pillow was wet.

What a horrible dream I had!

Thanks God, that it was only a dream!—A very bizarre dream, but it was only a dream, I

Realized—It has ended. Fortunately, it was over.

I was safe and in my bed, at my home. It was Friday morning.

Then, I heard the phone ringing.

I glanced at my watch—it was shortly before 6 a.m.—Who could call me so early?

Was it somebody calling me from Europe?—The time there was about 10 a.m.

I picked up the phone. I heard a voice of stranger -" May I talk to Mrs. Ryduchowski, please."

"I am Mrs. Ryduchowski,"—I answered—"Who are you? What do you want from me?"

"I am a nurse from the Saint Barnabas hospital,"-
the lady introduced herself.

She continued—"Your husband, Casimir…"

I have heard a short silence in the receiver, as if she
had hesitated about what should she be saying to me.

I had a thought—"Why is she calling me so early?"

Casimir, oh no, what was going on, there was
nothing wrong with him, it couldn't!

He was so well yesterday evening! He was so healthy!

But I felt a sudden fear.

I quickly asked the lady—"What is going on with
my husband?

How is he doing? Any problems?"

She sounded very assured when she answered my
question—"Your husband is doing fine now. He is
feeling fine. He had some minor problems, last night,
with urination. He was disconnected from the artificial bladder, last evening, and he couldn't urinate. He
probably had some hallucinations, all night, because
of this problem—he was calling your name several
times during the last night. He wanted to see you. He
asked us to call you immediately.

We didn't want to disturb your night's sleep; we
didn't want to wake you up so we have waited till the
morning. Your husband wants to talk to you, now."

"But, nurse,"—I asked—" How is he doing?"

"Oh, he is doing just fine,"—she answered—"We reconnected the artificial bladder to him and he is quite fine now. There is nothing to worry about!"

"Do you want to talk to your husband?"—she asked.

Soon, I heard Casimir's voice.

It sounded normal; like usual. I felt a sudden relief, and I heard a relief in his voice, too.

He was very calm, and sounded very realistic, when I heard him—"Danusia, I was absolutely sure that I would never see you again. Last night, I have had this bizarre out-of-the body experience, in which I had never believed before."

"I remember that I left my body. Danusia, I died the last night." —he continued.

"I had traveled,"—Casimir continued his story— "With an extremely high speed, through the outer space, to the another world!"

I remember I approached something like a large ceiling/cupola at the end of my journey. Then I saw both my parents, your father, all our relatives and friends who have already passed away! There were only dead people there. I even saw our friend Halinka!

They all were gathered behind the glass skylights in the ceiling and they were watching and smiling to me. I approached the skylight but I couldn't get through its opening. Then, I turned back, and returned back to my body.

I came back to my body!

I was back in my hospital bed!

There were nurses and doctors surrounding me. They were trying to rescue me!

I experienced this situation twice, during the last night.

The first time I was very scared.

I told to myself—"Oh no, oh God, I am not ready! I am not ready to die!"

I knew I was not prepared to die!

I didn't have my last communion! I couldn't die without taking my last communion!

I would like to take it!"—A visiting priest, I was later advised, asked my husband the prior morning if he would like to have a communion.

My husband wanted one, but the nurse didn't allow him to take it, since he was not allowed to take anything by mouth.

"The second time, I was ready to give up!"—My husband continued his story—

"I felt, that there was no sense to fight the destiny. If I had to die, I would do it now. I was relieved, I felt no sorry; everything would be over soon!

I was at a peace and quiet with myself!

I didn't feel any fear any longer.

I welcomed the end when I approached the skylight opening in the cupola.

But I was sent back, again. I came back again, to my body!

I did not die this time.

Danusia, could you please come to the hospital immediately!"—I heard a real urgency in his voice—"I am afraid, that if this bizarre experience happens to me again, I may never see you. I may never come back to you.

Please, hurry!"

CHAPTER V

IT IS SAFER TO TRAVEL BY A PLANE!

I felt a rush of an adrenaline in my body.

I knew my husband as a very skeptical, logically minded, individual and "I believe only in what I can see with my own eyes," person.

I could have never imagined him, having, and what is even stranger, reporting it to me any out-of the-body experiences!

Never! Not him!

Come on, everybody could have it but not he!

When I was sometimes talking to my friends, about some very bizarre, unexplained events, extra-terrestrial stories, and the out-of-the-body experiences that I read or heard about, he would always make jokes about these stories.

He would never believe in this kind of fantasy—he was always very materialistically minded.

He was atheist. Though he was frequently approached and invigilated, he had never expressed any slightest hesitation, and he always turned down any attempts made on him by the communist party recruiters in Poland.

With his talents and abilities, he was advised, he would "climb a ladder" and achieve a very high position and all connected to it privileges, if he only would agree to join the communist party.

However, he didn't want to "climb the ladder."

He didn't need all these privileges

He preferred to be a "free man."

However, frankly speaking, he also was not a religious person, not at all. He didn't attend

any masses in a church, unless on special occasions.

He has been more atteistically than spiritually, minded.

It was obvious to me, that he didn't believe in the existence of the spiritual world, souls, "another world's "existence, heaven, etc.

However, he also was not a "materialist"—he was never really interested in making money. He was not running after the material allures of our world.

It always I, who had to worry about our budget and how to meet the ends, in our family.

All he was really interested in was to be best in everything he was doing, and do the best and most honest work possible, in his field, at his job.

He always wanted to be a scientist.

I suspect that it was the main reason, the main propulsive force that has finally pushed us to the United States of America.

He was a very talented man, and in Poland, he has already made some significant scientific achievements, in the field of the fluid mechanics.

Frankly speaking, we both were doing quite well, in Poland, after we had graduated from the Technical University of Warsaw.

We had a nice apartment, good jobs, we even had a car (Yes, it was a real accomplishment to have a car in the "communist era" Poland and I will always remember this funny, East German made from plastic "Trabant" car.)

We started to travel extensively all over Europe. We were so called "yuppie" class.

Then, everything went "down the hill" in Poland.

We were sick and tired, of the communist, Mafia-type, regime. We knew that we would never be appreciated for what we were doing, without joining communist party.

We were tired of the sick economy.

We feared that due to our country's specific geographic location (Poland was surrounded by the" friendly neighbors," on its east and west borders—the former Soviet Union and East Germany), there would never be any hope for the political and economical improvement in our country.

We knew, that these "friendly" neighbors have already "helped," several times in the past, to kill freedom in Poland.

Poland was divided by Russians, Germans and Austrians into three parts at the end of the eighteen century, and ceased to exist, till the end of the First World War. There were several national uprisings, but they did not win the freedom for my country. Then, after a First World War, the freedom came finally.

My family was doing very well. They had big farms. Nobody was poor.

My father graduated just before the Second World War from the Warsaw University, as a forest engineer. He got very good and well paying job, as a forest manager, at the east part of Poland.

My aunt, a widow of the Polish Army colonel, became a "big fish." She got an exclusive license and became an independent manager of the wholesale operation for the stores distributing alcoholic beverages at the east part of Poland. She went to Baranovicze town, and my mother has joined her.

They were young, beautiful, and they were rich.

The world belonged to them.

Then, the Second World War had changed everything. The "friendly neighbors,"—German and Russian nazis, both invaded Poland in September of 1939.

Again, innocent people were killed in my country. The evil had triumphed, again.

However, my parents (who haven't met yet), were luckier.

My father was warned, in an advance, by his tailor (who later was disclosed as a Russian collaborator), that as a Polish engineer, and as a member of an "intelligent elite," he was on a "special" list, and would be deported to Siberia, Russia, for a certain extinction.

My father managed to escape to a capital of Poland, Warsaw (this city later became a "German General Province" under German occupation), and worked at a factory, doing a manual job, during the entire Second World War.

The German Nazis, almost executed him on one occasion, and only due to the extremely strange and happy circumstances (he was set free by a German soldier, whose father was also a forest engineer, on an impulse of sympathy), he survived the war.

My mother and her sister were also advised by some friends to "run away" from Russian Nazis, and managed to escape from Baranowicze town to Warsaw.

My parents met and spent the entire Second World Wartime in Warsaw.

I still remember the horror stories, told by them, about their personal experiences to which they were exposed, during the Second World War.

Then, a war was over and the "freedom" came—but shortly after the end of the war, my father was approached to join a communist party. Since he did not want to collaborate with communists, shortly after his refusal he was accused of a collaboration with the "rebels"(In fact, these "rebels" were soldiers of the Independent Polish Army, who were hiding from communists in the forest, supervised by my father.)

As a result of this accusation, my father was imprisoned and hardly avoided a death sentence. When he left the prison finally he was, according to my mother, practically an invalid- quite a different person he was when he first met my mother.

My husband's father had to hide from Germans (under manure, in a stable) for the entire Second World War time, only for one reason; he was a Polish teacher. As such person, he automatically was sentenced to death.

With these experiences in our families, we thought that things would never be better in Poland. There would always be "troubles" in our country and "good neighbors" will always" help" us to stay imprisoned under some kind of a regime.

Poland would always be sacrificed by its allies, and attacked first, if there were any adverse developments in the world's politics. There would be nobody to help.

"There has to be a better place, somewhere else, on our earth, than our country, "—we thought—"A free world full of promise."

We were young, talented, and not scared to do any work.

"There had to be a place in our world where you could fulfill all your dreams. Be appreciated for who you are."—we dreamt.

Feeling that we would never be allowed to achieve what we wanted, unless we join the communist party, we were eager to try our luck somewhere else.

I have applied for and I got an unexpected and almost "against all odds," contract at the University in Nigeria.

I was offered a Senior Lecturer's position, good salary and benefits, and a chance to see a different world.

Africa!

I would never have a chance to see this exotic world, to see its nature and the people,

unless I go there!

I went to Nigeria on May 5th, 1981. I was a Senior Lecturer there. My first lecture, in English, was on a "rock blasting techniques", ha!

Soon, my husband has joined me.

I helped him to get a job at the same University, as a Senior Lecturer

We were both lecturing, and my husband became actively involved in a theoretical and applied research on the alternative energy sources—solar energy applications.

He invented a very efficient solar pump to be used in under developed countries, and an innovative, solar powered air-conditioning system.

He wrote several scientific/technical articles on this topic.

He published these articles in the recognized journals worldwide.

At this time (the beginning of the eighties), the crude oil's price was going up, skyrocketing and the cost of energy was increasing. He hoped that his solar energy systems would help people save energy! He believed that his solar energy systems were a future for developing countries. He was very enthusiastic about his research!

We stayed in Nigeria for approximately two and half years.

We were doing quite well there, and I believe that we both were liked and appreciated by our black students and colleagues. Also, with two salaries (housing, electricity, etc., were free), we were living quite nicely, and a good exchange rate of naira (local currency) to the US dollar was helping to our well—being.

We were living at a beautiful campus, designed and built by the Italian architects. We had a large house, a house boy, and a gardener. We could travel everywhere, both in Africa and worldwide. We even came on a six weeks' vacation to the United States, in 1982. We did an extensive four-week sightseeing, by a Greyhound bus, of the United States. We even saw Las Vegas and the Great Canyon!

Meanwhile, things were not turning better in our home country, Poland.

Suddenly, the martial law was introduced in Poland on December 13, 1981. My country was endangered again. Our "friendly neighbors" did not want to allow for any freedom in Poland. The "Solidarity" movement went underground. It appeared that the communist regime would be in power forever. The borders were closed, and the international travel possibilities were available for only a few "lucky ones."

Practically, all the international travel was postponed, for Polish people—to the "East" (Eastern Europe coalition) they became the rebels, to the "West"(NATO countries) they were poor refugees who have to be fed on the expense of local taxpayers.

Frankly speaking, we were afraid, as an entire family, to travel for a vacation to Poland. We could never get passports for all of us, again, from a martial law regime.

The communists could keep one or more of us, as a "hostage" (This was a common practice, at this time in Poland; not to allow the entire family to travel together— in this way, the " danger" of an escape of the "slaves" was less possible.)

Meantime, in Nigeria, a time for the governmental elections was approaching. The two main political parties were actively fighting with each other for a power.

The supporters of these parties were also fighting with each other. We started to see houses being burnt, motor vehicles overturned and burnt on the roads.

Yes, it was getting more and more dangerous there.

Martial law in Nigeria was a question of weeks, maybe days.

Though we liked this country, its beautiful nature, and friendly and open Nigerian people, we couldn't stay there any longer.

I was not feeling well in Nigeria—the climate was too hot and humid, and I have already had several malaria attacks.

Each attack made me weaker—I was allergic to the anti- malaria medicines. I couldn't take it for a longer period of time, without feeling sick.

We didn't want to go back to Poland because of the political situation there. We felt that there was no future for us in Poland, and we feared that since we both belonged to the "Solidarity" movement, which became illegal under the martial law in Poland, we could face some kind of prosecution.

Also, there was no future for us in Nigeria. We saw that loss of democracy in this country was a question of time. Also, an increasing corruption was making it more difficult to live there. We started to hear about robberies on some " foreigners" (In fact, one of our friends was killed in a robbery in his house in Ibadan, shortly after we left Nigeria.)

Meanwhile, my husband got an invitation from the University of Miami, USA.

His scientific paper on the solar energy system was accepted for a presentation, and he was invited to deliver it at the 6th International Conference on the Alternative Energy Sources in Miami.

We made a quick decision; we would go to the United States. We would try "our luck" there. For sure, there will be good opportunities for an expert on the alternate energy sources, and for a civil/structural engineer, both with the Ph.D. degrees.

We wanted to do research, and for sure, there was no better place to do an applied research, than the United States of America!

"If things do not turn as well as we expected,"—we speculated,—"we can always immigrate to another place on our earth such as, for example, Canada or Australia."

I do not want to elaborate here on a detailed description of our experiences, since our arrival to the United States of America.

It is a story for another book!

Maybe, one day, I will sit down, and write about some of our adventures, but not now!

Now, we are where we are.

Let's say we are a middle class Americans. We are both American citizens.

And one of us just has had this extraordinary, out-of-the-body, experience!

Do not pull my leg! No kidding!

We are both engineers—we are both scientifically and analytically minded!

We believe only in material things that can be designed by an engineer—we believe in the achievements of a modern civilization!

We do not believe in anything that cannot be seen! No ghosts! We are materialists!

Space traveling, why not? But to travel out-of-the body? Never!

We can travel, for sure—but only in a spaceship!

Even better, eventually, why not to travel in an airplane?

After all, it is much safer to fly in an airplane, then in a spaceship!

CHAPTER VI

WHAT WENT WRONG
THIS NIGHT?

I knew that things went wrong, somewhere, and something really bad had happened to my husband last night at the hospital.

I would have to go to the hospital, immediately!

I must find out, and help my husband!

I awakened my son, Michael,—"Wake up! Get ready! Your daddy has just called me telling that he was probably dying—there is no time to waste, we have to hurry!"

I was in a state of panic—what has been happening to my husband?

What was the reason for such a sudden deterioration of his health?

He was in such a good shape last evening—he only had a slight hick-up, from the repositioned tube irritating his throat, but otherwise, he was feeling great!

We were talking about his homecoming at the end of the week- maybe on Sunday?

I called my husband's doctor; Doctor F. It was 6 a.m. —I got his answering service. He answered my emergency call in the five minutes time.

I almost yelled at him—"How dare, how dare you, doctor, what had been done to my husband? I left him feeling so well last evening, and during the last night, he almost passed away!

Doctor, what is your excuse, your explanation, please?"

The doctor was very calm. He didn't want to answer, right away. He advised that he needed some time to find out, what had happened to my husband, last night.

He would call me back.

He did, in a few minutes time.

His story was a simple one—my husband was disconnected from the artificial bladder, last night. He couldn't urinate (Usually, I do not remember that my husband used to have a frequent urge to urinate during the night time—he could last all night without going to the bathroom, not like me!) He started to hallucinate. He was reconnected to the artificial bladder, and again, he was fine. I shouldn't worry.

There was no need for me to worry. It was a simple problem. It was solved satisfactorily.

Everything would be fine.

The doctor would stay in a touch with the hospital. Also, he was going to see my husband early in the morning (The doctor was having another operation at the hospital, in the morning.)

The doctor's explanation was a very realistic one.

He was very supportive, and he answered, surpassingly quickly, to my worried call.

I felt that my husband was in a good doctor's hands.

Then, I heard from the doctor, an advice, that I would always remember—

"You have to be strong! You will not help your husband, if you loose control of yourself. If you really want to help him, never panic! You have to be calm!"

I immediately understood the true meaning of these words.

So, when I finally entered my husband's hospital room, after over one-hour trip in the terrible traffic jam on a Garden State Parkway, I was calm, quiet, and organized.

I knew that I couldn't afford to be hysterical!

I smiled broadly to him—"What is going on with you, old boy, a small problem, you couldn't "pee of", and you made such a big noise?"

He looked almost normal, slightly pale, but he was conscious, when he answered—

"I do not know, what had happened to me last night, Danusia.

I can't understand it. I feel sorry for all this mess I made, last night. I remember, I called you, I called your name, several times. I was asking for you entire night, but you didn't come." (I couldn't come because nobody has called me.)

He continued—"Danusia, I had such a bizarre experience, last night. First, I remember that I heard a beautiful music, and while listening to this music, I saw a movie. In this movie, I went back through my entire life.

The events that were revived in my memory, in this movie, were records from my entire life's experiences. But only the best moments, the moments full of joy and happiness, were replayed in this movie!

These were Christmas parties at my home and I was so happy to get my favorite toys; these were games with my childhood favorite friends, I laughed and played them again; and the parties at my parents' house; their anniversaries and celebrations.

Danusia till now, I didn't realize that I had such a happy and worry free childhood!

And during all this time, I heard this beautiful music. I do not know who composed it. I must find it out, when I am well again. I must find and buy all these wonderful musical records.

Then, after the movie from my entire life ended, I suddenly left my body. I was traveling through a space, a space full of colorful lights, at an incredibly high speed."

My husband smiled and he looked at me,—

"At the beginning of my travel, I remember that I was very suprised. I didn't know what was going on with me! What was happening to me? Suddenly, I understood. I left my body. I died.

I remember that at the end of my space journey, I approached the "end" of the space. I was traveling towards—it was like an immense, endless cupola, with curved walls and a ceiling. There were round openings in this ceiling, similar to the skylights. Behind these skylights, I saw numerous faces. There were people behind the glass, and they were watching me. They were smiling to Me."—he continued.

"I saw my parents, my Uncle Frank, your aunts, your father Franek, my grandparents. I even saw our friends—Halinka (who died of cancer three years ago, at age 39), and Thaddeus (who died of a heart attack two years ago.)

I saw all the people I knew—but there were only the people, who have already passed away. There were no people whom I knew to be alive.

"These were only dead people, Danusia",—my husband told seriously—" I couldn't approach them. I couldn't get through the skylight."

Then, I traveled back to my body. I was back in my bed, in this hospital.

"This experience has happened twice to me, during the last night"—he continued—

"I remember, that during the time I was "back" in my bed, the hospital staff was rescuing me. During my awakening, I remember that I was reconnected to the artificial bladder. I remember the doctors telling me that I was hallucinating, because of problems with an artificial bladder and lack of urination.

I remember, that I was also talking to the doctors and nurses, and I pretended that everything was all right with me, that nothing wrong was happening to me."—he continued.

"I even remember that I fluently spoke several foreign languages, languages which I do not have any command, or which I know only slightly, when I am conscious. I remember that I fluently spoke German, French, and even Russian to the hospital staff."

My husband looked at me. He was very serious, and his chin was shaking—"Dana, I am ashamed of myself. I do not remember everything, but I am afraid that I probably could be telling some nonsense to these people around me.

These people, the hospital staff, and another patient in my room, they can laugh at me, now!"—he looked really upset.

"How stupid, how stupid of me it was, to be so totally out of control, talking some kind of nonsense, which I do not even can remember now!"

I listened to my husband patiently.

I tried to reassure him that nobody would laugh at him, because of his last night's talkativeness.

Nobody should laugh at such a sick person.

But meantime, I had some second thoughts.

I thought—"What was the reason, what was really happening to my husband during the last night?

What could have happened, why has he had all these bizarre hallucinations?"

Frankly speaking, I couldn't believe, and I still have doubts that he really had all these out-of-the-body experiences.

I took his report as a fantastic story, something that could not have ever happened in reality. It was really nonsense!

But, what was really happening to him, since I left him last evening, and he was feeling so well? What was a reason for such a sudden deterioration?

Slowly, a full story of the last night's events, from the beginning of the night (after I left the hospital), to the moment when I was called by a hospital nurse at 6 a.m. in the morning, was disclosed by my husband.

He was taken out from the morphine, late last afternoon.

In the late evening, after I went back home, he heard that another patient in his room was asking for a painkiller.

My husband was feeling fine, and he didn't really feel any major pain, he told me, but after he heard this another patient's request, he thought that it would be good, as a preventive measure, to get a painkiller—just to prevent the perspective pain. He asked a nurse for a painkiller.

"How stupid of me it was, Danusia, but after I heard him asking for a painkiller, I also wanted one.

I remember, that a nurse, whom I had never seen at the hospital before (she was wearing a red dress, she was not wearing a hospital uniform), gave me an intravenous injection, saying that it was a painkiller I requested.

Soon after I received it, some strange developments started to happen to me. My heart started to beat erratically, like crazy!

This situation has never happened to me before!

I feared, that my heart would jump out from my chest!"—he continued.

"My heart was beating faster and stronger!—Its natural rhythm was totally disrupted!

Soon, I felt dizzy. Then, I had all these "hallucinations", such as the out-of-the-body experience, which I have already reported to you"—my husband looked at me—

"Danusia, I suspect that this painkiller might have caused my last night's problems!

It was not a problem with the urination—I just didn't have any urge to urinate. I always can sleep for the entire night, without urinating. Usually, I do not have to go to the bathroom during the nighttime. I almost never do it! It was not the problem with urination—it was a painkiller's reaction, "—he sounded as if he were afraid of something—

"Without this painkiller, this entire situation wouldn't have happened. Without it, or if I were given another painkiller, all these last night's problems wouldn't have happened.

Danusia, I suspect that if it were not for my strong and healthy heart (my husband had never had any heart problems), I would have died, last night!"

He sounded very uneasy—"I am very lucky, that my heart survived all this strain, this unusual, erratically beating!"

Danusia, maybe it sounds very stupid, but I am really scared of staying at the hospital alone! I cannot be left alone or you will never see me again.

He continued—"Also, I am somehow scared of this nurse. She looked so strangely at me, while giving me this painkiller. I am scared that she can give me this painkiller, again.

Danusia, you have to stay with me, at my bed in the hospital, day and night, until I feel well again."

He looked around—" I still have some hallucinations (not similar to these previously described in the out-of-the-body experience)—I hear some voices. I know that there is nobody around me but you; but I hear some other people talking around me!

You should stay with me and watch what kind of a medication I am given. I do not want to be given the same painkiller again!"

He sounded really scared—"If you leave me alone, I am afraid that I will not survive the next night! I am scared! Help me, please!"

I have listened to my husband very skeptically. I could not believe that any painkiller might have caused these problems!

However, I was anxious to learn what kind of painkiller it could have been? What medication was given to my husband last night?

I went to check it with a nurse.

She reviewed my husband's records.

"Your husband has asked for a painkiller, himself, and he was given one,"—she advised. "According to the records, the night crew doctor advised that your husband be given a painkiller."

"What was he given, nurse?"—I asked—" What is the name of this painkiller?"

"He was given the Demerol"—the nurse advised.

I continued to interrogate her—"Did my husband request this specific painkiller?

Did he ask for Demerol? I have never heard about this medication before, nurse!"

She answered—"Oh no, he didn't ask for Demerol specifically, but it is a very popular medication, and an effective painkiller, and we give it usually to the patients who are in a serious pain.

This medication acts very quickly, and alleviates pain considerably!"—she answered.

"Yes, nurse, but my husband started to feel very sick after he was administered this medication, his heart started to beat erratically, he got extremely strong heart palpitations and then he had extremely bizarre hallucinations!"—I continued—

"He just told me that he had died, he passed away, and saw some members of our family and friends, whom we knew not to be alive any longer.

These kind of hallucinations have never happened to him before, nurse!"

"Oh, yes,"—the nurse has smiled—" Demerol can cause severe hallucinations, sometimes, in some patients, allergic to it. It can have such a side effect, in some people that are allergic to it, and probably your husband belongs to them. But there is nothing really to worry about; everything is under control now. Your husband was feeling very well during the entire last night, we were watching him, and he is fine now."—she replied—

"I will write it down that your husband is allergic to Demerol, so he will not be given it, next time, when he requests a painkiller."

"Thank you, nurse"—I was very grateful to her. I knew that a really nice and cooperative hospital staff was taking a good care of my husband.

I believed that without their help my husband wouldn't get well.

The hospital staff was taking good care of him, and I was confident, that my husband was in "good hands".

"Casimir, he is probably allergic to this medication, to this Demerol!"—I realized what was the problem.

"There were no hallucinations, no out-of-the-body experiences. It was just a common allergy."—Allergy is a much easier problem to understand, than these bizarre out-of-the body travels, isn't it?

After I finished interviewing the nurse, I went back to my husband. I calmed him down—"You were hysterical, Casimir, the painkiller you were given, this painkiller sometimes caused bizarre hallucinations in some people who were allergic to it!

Your experiences were quite normal, according to the nurse's advise, to most people who are allergic to this painkiller after they get it! A nurse wrote down that you were allergic to this medication. This medication would never be given to you again."

(Later on we always advised medical staff about my husband's allergy to Demerol, on every occasion.)

But my husband has looked at me with such unbelieving eyes—" But what about my heart, my heart problems, this erratical, irregular beating, extremely strong heart palpitations. I was sure, sometimes, that my heart would jump out of my chest, then, it was stopping suddenly. I have never had such exordinary heart problems, such a disruption of my heart rhythm, in my entire life!"

"Oh, Casimir,"—I answered him—"You are exaggerating!"

"You did not have any real heart problems, last night—these were just common allergy symptoms, according to the nurse advise!"—I smiled.

"Also, you have just imagined, yourself, all these bizarre out-of-the-body experiences—these hallucinations were simply due to your allergic reaction to this painkilling medication, to the Demerol, which you were administered."

However, deeply inside, I was not satisfied with the nurse's answer.

"Why,"—I thought,—" If they knew that some people can be allergic to Demerol, that this medication may cause some severe, adverse, allergic effects, such as hallucinations, etc., why this medication is given to the sick people?

Why my husband has got it?

Why this particular drug was administered to him?

Why not a Tylenol, in a suppository form, or another similar painkiller, that doesn't cause such a bizarre "allergy" was given to him?"

But, at the time of my husband's stay at the hospital, I didn't know yet about side effects which the Demerol when combined with the narcotics, for example, a morphine, had caused in some other patients.

Later on, I read some horror stories. I read articles in the newspapers such as the New York Times that very strange and sudden deaths have occurred after Demerol was administered to the patients who were under the influence of narcotics, such, as for an example, the morphine. I have read a story about a nineteen year old girl, admitted to one of the New York City hospitals, with some unusual symptoms (later on, it was found out that she was on "drugs"), who was given the Demerol. Though otherwise healthy, she had died of a sudden heart attack, at this hospital, shortly after Demerol was administered to her. A presence of narcotics was later discovered in her blood, during the post-mortem. Her family was suing the hospital, for negligence in her death.

Also, I have read in The New York Times a story that a nurse (to Ms. Doris Duke, a billionaire), had certified in the court that a high dose of morphine and then a Demerol, were administered to this heiress, on the night of her death.

I believe that I remember reading this nurse's statement that doctors informed her on the late evening, that the patient wouldn't survive till the morning.

All these deaths were under legal investigation in the courts, according to the newspaper's relations.

In all these cases, a common fact was that the Demerol was administered to the people who were under the influence of the narcotics. They died shortly after receiving it. They died of a heart attack. My husband was still under the influence of morphine, when he was given Demerol!

I cannot believe that this medication was given to him or to any of the above patients, on special purpose/knowingly (To cause a harm to him or other patients.)

I can't imagine that there could be anybody in the medical establishment, any doctor, or medical staff, who would with a full conscience, and without his/her patient's consent, cause such a harm to any patient.

However, in my opinion, somebody should make a thorough investigation about the adverse effects of

Demerol, and the administration of this medication should be evaluated in each case, so it would be never again administered to the patients who, like my husband, were under the influence of narcotics!

Fortunately, my husband has survived this (pain) killing experience!

CHAPTER VII

A DEATH SENTENCE

Since my husband was too scared to stay at the hospital alone, I decided to stay at his bedside, day and night, until he is well again.

I stayed at his bed for the next three or four nights, with an exception for very short, 3 to 4 hours, breaks for going home to have a shower, and a short rest. (Our son Michael stayed with him, when I was gone.)

During the nighttime, sitting in a chair at his bedside I watched him sleeping and during the day, I talked to him, about everything what I could think and talk about.

I tried to entertain him with my stories.

I was often repeating my stories, sometimes stupid, while I was talking. These stories had only one important meaning—I wanted him to forget about all his "hallucinations."

I wanted him to forget about his fear and get him "back" to the normal world.

I also wanted to talk, so I myself could forget about my own fears, and fears about his health condition.

Soon after I arrived to the hospital (on Friday morning, immediately after receiving an urgent call from my husband), I met for the first time in person doctor F.

A short and balding man in his fifties, he entered my husband's room where I, and our son Michael, were sitting at his bedside.

When he saw my husband and us, he smiled to my husband—" Oh, I see you have visitors today, your son and daughter, are visiting you, Mr. Ryduchowski.

You are a lucky man, today!"

I have approached doctor F.—"Doctor, I am Casimir's wife, I called you this morning.

What is going on with my husband, doctor, please? He had such bizarre hallucinations, last night!"

Doctor looked at me—" Sorry, I thought you were Casimir's daughter. Everything is fine

with your husband, he is doing fine.

As I told you on the phone, the problems with his urination have caused some deterioration of your husband health, he couldn't urinate, last night. He was disconnected from an artificial bladder too early."

Doctor F. checked my husband's chart, and had examined him.

After I saw doctor F., I felt a rush of hope, and a confidence that everything would be well with my husband, since he was under care of such a good doctor.

Doctor F. made a very good impression on me—after seeing him, I was sure that every disease, including cancer, will go away, after this doctor starts treating my husband.

I talked to doctor F. several times; on each occasion when he was "inspecting" my husband.

According to the doctor's advise, a cancerous growth, less than 1 inch in diameter, was found on the head of my husband's pancreas. This growth was pushing on the bile duct, hindering a flow of the bile from the liver. This cancerous growth was removed, together with portions of the pancreas, stomach, and intestines surrounding pancreas, during the operation.

The good news was that no cancerous growths were found on my husband's liver or other organs nearby.

The lymph nodes in the vicinity of the pancreas were also removed, during the operation, and were sent to the laboratory for an analysis.

According to the doctor, the operation was successful, and if only cancer hadn't metastasized to the lymph nodes (what would be found through the laboratory tests), the prognosis for my husband recovery was very good.

I was waiting for the laboratory tests' result to come, every day.

Finally, they arrived.

The doctor wanted to talk to me.

I met him in the corridor, outside of my husband's hospital room.

I saw from doctor's face, that he had very important news for me.

He began—" Mrs. Ryduchowski, I got the results of the laboratory tests of your husband lymph nodes. As I told you before, the cancerous growth on his pancreas was relatively small, and it was removed during the operation.

Unfortunately, the laboratory tests have shown that the cancer had already metastasized to the lymph nodes—in fact, the cancer cells were found in all the lymph nodes tested."

I interrupted the doctor impatiently—" Doctor, what is the outlook? You mentioned that cancerous growth was relatively small, and it didn't attack the liver, etc., yet? That my husband's organs were free from cancer?"

Doctor F. looked at me with a sad expression on his face.

I understood that he felt very compassionate towards both my husband and me.

"Unfortunately, Mrs. Ryduchowski, the outlook for your husband's future is not good. Not good at all!

If the cancer were confined to the head of the pancreas only, we would be positively sure, that it had been entirely removed during the operation.

But, once it metastasizes to the lymph nodes, it practically travels all over the body systems. It can metastasize and start growing again somewhere else—and it usually does, within a very short time span."

He looked very sad—"Your husband was not freed from cancer during the operation. Practically, since the cancer has already spread to the lymph nodes, he still has this extremely malignant cancer."

"Unfortunately, I have a very bad news for you, Mrs. Ryduchowski—usually, the patients diagnosed with the pancreatic cancer that had already metastasized to the lymph nodes, have very poor chance even for the two years survival.

I am very sorry, Mrs. Ryduchowski, that I have to tell it to you, but I think that you should be prepared for the worst possible happening—your husband's death in the very near future."

"Any help, doctor?"—I begged.

"Any modern, miraculous medication, some new developments in medicine, which can

help save my husband life?

How can I help him?—I don't want him to die!

I love him, I need him—our children need him, too!"

Doctor F. looked at me with compassion—I knew that he would have preferred to tell me

good news instead of the bad one.

I knew that he felt really sorry, having to say only the bad news.

I knew that he really wanted to help us. I am still very grateful to him, and I appreciate his expertise, and honesty, in warning me as to the seriousness of my husband's disease.

"There is always a hope,"—the doctor said—"There is a good, modern hospital in Manhattan, the Memorial Sloan-Kettering Cancer Center Hospital. I have heard that they were very advanced in the cancer treatments. There is a new drug, called Taxol. Maybe the experts at this hospital would be able to help your husband, though, as I far as I know, there is no conventional treatment, no medication effectively working against the metastasized pancreatic cancer, currently."

I interrupted him—"Doctor, I think that my husband should visit this hospital. We can't wait till the cancer further spreads, appears and grows somewhere else. We have to fight it before it shows up again!

Could you, please, refer us to this hospital?"

Doctor F., the surgeon, smiled at me patiently—"I can't refer your husband to this hospital now. I can only refer him to the oncologist. I know very good oncologist, who can possibly help your husband. He may refer him to this hospital."

I felt a rush of hope—" When, doctor, when, can my husband see this oncologist?

I want him to get started, as soon as possible, on this miraculous cancer treatment!"

"First, your husband must get well after the operation. Then, he would be able to see the oncologist"—Doctor F advised.

"The oncologist will assure that your husband gets the best suitable treatment, currently available. If needed, he would refer him to the Memorial Sloan-Kettering Cancer Center. I can not make these recommendations."—doctor F., the surgeon, advised.

I thanked the doctor, and I went back to see my husband.

"What are the news?"—He asked,—"You look so pale, you have tears in your eyes!"

What doctor F. did tell you? Did you hear any bad news from him, didn't you?"

"Oh no, I am just very tired, after so many days and nights of staying in the hospital,"—I lied. I had to be strong, I had to be strong, no crying!

Be a strong woman, Danusia!

"I am so tired, that I am really a nervous wreck. The doctor gave me great news, the tumor that was removed from your pancreas was really small and no new cancerous growths were found on the surrounding organs. He told me that he would refer you for a further preventive treatment to the oncologist, after you get better. You would need, on a preventive basis, further treatment. You will be well, after this treatment is completed, I am sure."

Then, I realized that I wouldn't be able to make these lies any longer.

I excused myself, and I run to the ladies' room.

I started to cry and I cried for a long time.

When I finally calmed down, I put a lot of powder on my face, a new layer of mascara on my eyelashes, a thick layer of lipstick, and with a face painted like a clown, I went back to entertain my husband.

However, he found from the expression on my face, that I was hiding something, maybe some bad news, from him. He told me that I was looking tired.

This coming night, he advised, he would be able to stay alone in the hospital—he was feeling well enough. I was not needed any longer.

He wanted me to go home and have some rest.

He advised me that I needed to rest and I was also needed at home, since our children

didn't see me for quite a long time.

So, I went back home—I kept visiting him at the hospital on late afternoons, every day.

He spent several more days, about a week or more in the hospital (altogether he stayed at the hospital approximately for the two weeks' time), and then he came back home.

I remember driving him home and how happy we were to be together again!

It was Saturday, a day before Sunday Easter.

A great day to be back home!

He had to stay in the bed at home and a health aide was visiting him, cleaning his difficult to heal wound with the hydrogen peroxide, on a daily basis.

This wound was badly infected and it was difficult to heal. One day, it was closing and on another day, it was reopening again. We had a feeling, that it would be never healed.

He also had to take, for a certain time, antibiotics for the bladder infection caused probably by the emergency re-connection of the artificial bladder at the hospital, during the night when he had all these "hallucinations".

But he was at home—at last, we were all home together, and there were also good news coming from the outside world. He got pay—raise, when he was at the hospital. He also got numerous fruit baskets, and flowers, from the friendly coworkers at his workplace.

His friends were calling, to support him. He was liked and admired by most people working with him.

Physically, he felt sometimes better and sometimes worse. Soon after coming back home, he got a high fever, over 103 F. This fever stayed for a long time, over three weeks.

We called doctor F. for help. He requested a blood test, which didn't indicate on an enlarged number of the white cell count in his blood caused by an infection.

We were advised that it was not an infection that caused this fever.

We felt that a new dose of antibiotics might help to fight it.

We called Doctor F. Again, this very wise doctor advised us: "Mr. Ryduchowski, you should try to stay away from the antibiotics as far away as possible. If used needlessly (when there was no infection), or if used too often, they will be of no help when they are really needed. The bacteria and viruses are becoming resistant to most of the antibiotics. The antibiotics would not work in a real need."

However, my husband was given a prescription for the antibiotics. He could buy and use them only if the fever would stay for longer than two days; since his recent call to the doctor's office. However, fortunately my husband has never needed to take these prescribed but forbidden to him antibiotics—the fever has disappeared on its own, and without any antibiotics' usage.

My husband started to feel great!

In a six-week time since operation, he returned back to work.

However, he still had problems with healing of his wound which, though treated with the hydrogen peroxide, was partially closing sometimes and then reopening again.

For the first time I saw an effectiveness of the "alternative treatment".

My sister has sent him a special bee propolis ointment from Poland.

This stubbornly reopening wound was healed almost in no time, after this ointment was applied to it!

Finally feeling well, my husband made an appointment to see an oncologist, Doctor M.

Doctor M. also asked me to attend this first visit at his office.

The oncologist was a very busy person. We had to wait for him for more than one hour, before he showed up.

"I am glad, I am glad,"—he advised,—"That both of you, Mr. And Mrs. Ryduchowski, were able to come to see me."

"It is very important, that both of you understand the seriousness of your situation."

"What kind of treatment will you prescribe to my husband, doctor,"—I interrupted.

"What is the outlook, the chance, for my husband's survival?"

The doctor moved in his chair nervously.

"Frankly speaking, Mr. and Mrs. Ryduchowski, there is presently no known medical treatment, that was found to be effective against metastasized pancreatic cancer."

"I want to be frank and open about it,"—the doctor advised.

"Currently, there is no medication to be proven successful against the metastasized pancreatic cancer, the type of cancer your husband has got.

The statistics is very unfavorable in this case. Less than 10% of patients survive first two years, and less than 5% survive five years since the diagnosis and operation of this type of cancer."

"But doctor, there has to be some help; we were told by doctor F. about this famous Memorial Sloan-Kettering Cancer Center in Manhattan. Maybe the experts at this hospital can help us?"—I begged.

"Oh no,"—the doctor answered,—" I am very much updated in the cancer treatments. The experts at this hospital do not have yet any proven treatment effective against pancreatic cancer."

"They can offer you some experimental treatments, for sure.

But, I want to be frank with you. I do not want anybody to make experiments on you, Mr. Ryduchowski.

I wouldn't advise you to let anybody to experiment on your husband in his present health condition, Mrs. Ryduchowski.

If your condition, Mr. Ryduchowski, deteriorates considerably, I would advise you to consider some kind of experimental treatment. At least, you can contribute, in this way, to the development of the medical sciences."

He continued—"The only treatment I would like to advise you presently, Mr. Ryduchowski, is a light chemotherapy and radiation treatment. At least, this treatment would not cause too many harms to you.

Frankly speaking, Mr. Ryduchowski, I want to tell you, that there is no chemotherapy treatment found to be effective against the pancreatic cancer.

The chemotherapy, which would be applied to you, Mr. Ryduchowski, should make the radiation treatment more effective. It means, that you pancreas would be more responsive to the radiation treatment."

"Will this radiation treatment help my husband, doctor?"—I asked.

"There was almost no research done on the effectiveness of this combined chemotherapy and radiation treatment, frankly speaking,"—doctor M. advised.

"A survey made on a very limited group of patients, revealed that this treatment had prolonged life of about 35% of the patients surveyed to about two years.

In other words, it was found, that about 35% of patients treated, survived up to two years after this treatment.

But I want you to know that this survey was made on a very limited group of patients,"—the doctor advised.

"What has happened with the 35% of patients who survived two years? How long did they live later on?"—I asked.

The doctor continued—"It doesn't mean that the people who underwent this treatment, were cured from cancer totally and became healthy.

It only means that 35% of the patients from the treated group survived up to two years, while only 10% of the untreated patients from a comparable group survived for a similar time.

I want you to understand that this treatment doesn't guarantee that you will survive two years, Mr. Ryduchowski. Cancer of the pancreas (Pancreatic Carcinoma) is one of the most malignant, if not the most malignant, cancers.

The prognosis is very serious, for the patients diagnosed with this kind of cancer.

Do you want to undergo this treatment, anyhow, Mr. Ryduchowski?"

"Yes, yes, doctor, I do,"—my husband answered.

"35% vice 10% chance, it sounds like a big difference to me."

I heard a hope in his voice—" Why not to go for it? I am ready to try!"

I understood that he wanted to live longer than only up to two years, since his operation.

I decided to fight for his life!

To me, a statement that only 35% patients (of a very small, representative sample of about twenty patients) survived up to two years, with the quality of their life being impaired by a fear, and sickness, sounded like a death sentence.

I didn't want to take a chance that my husband would share a fate of the remaining 65%, of the less "lucky" patients.

I didn't want to take chance that after two years of a miserable life, full of fear, maybe he will be still alive, but his life will be more resembling a life of a vegetable than of an active human being!

I decided to do something, on my own, to help my husband.

I decided to say "no" to this death sentence!

CHAPTER VIII

HOW I BECAME A "WITCH DOCTOR"

Soon, my husband underwent a six weeks' radiation treatment at the Saint Barnabas Radiological Center. A five-day stay at the hospital preceded this treatment, where he received an intravenous chemotherapy treatment.

Meantime, I started to do a research on my own, into the alternative cancer treatments.

I bought or borrowed every available book, which was dealing on this topic. I was becoming an expert on the alternative cancer treatments.

I started to feel that there was a hope!

One of my husband's friends at his office, a coworker, advised my husband about the beneficial effect of the Pau D'Arco herb.

This friend had a history of the bladder cancer himself and after five years since his operation (during which time he was on the Pau D'Arco treatment), his doctors diagnosed him as a cancer-free.

I researched on every information about properties of the Pau D'Arco herb and I became very enthusiastic about this herb.

Soon, my husband was started on the Pau D'Arco treatment—he was even drinking it, during his chemotherapy treatment at the hospital (in a smaller quantity than at home), and he felt very well during this chemotherapy.

We bought the Pau D'Arco extract, as recommended by his coworker, at one of the health food stores in Newark, NJ.

My husband has recommended this extract to another patient, sharing hospital room with him. Although this patient was diagnosed with a terminal cancer; I saw a hope rising in his eyes, after he learned about this Pau D'Arco treatment.

Soon, the health food store in Newark has run out of the supply of the Pau D'Arco extract—then, we were advised that its manufacture be suspended.

It was a big problem for us (This extract was imported from Brazil). I decided to make this extract myself. My husband drunk it 3 times daily and he claimed that "my" extract was even better (I used a Pau D'Arco bark supplied by very reputable vendors), tasted much better, and was probably safer (no preservatives were added to this herb) and it could be even more efficient, than the extract which we had previously bought in the health food store in Newark. My husband loved it!

At the same time, I experienced a happening that I considered a coincidence, but a very bizarre coincidence—I have found in the "The Bottom Line" magazine, an information about a special report on the mind/body power, written by a cancer survivor, Mr. Harry De Camp. I decided to order this report, and by a very bizarre coincidence, it has arrived after at least two weeks' waiting time, just on the first day of my husband's arrival to the hospital. First, I reviewed this report myself (I didn't want my husband to read one of these very scientific and "sophisticated", but somehow not upraising, or even depressing, books on a mind/body power, but I wanted him to read something that was really uplifting, and optimistic.)

After reading it, I decided to bring this report to the hospital, and I convinced my husband to read it.

He previously turned down all my attempts on advising him "proper" books for reading. While I had a large library of health books on the alternative medicine, and I tried to " drop " them at the most convenient places for him to read, he almost never turned a page. He just ignored these books and never acknowledged the information they contained. Instead, he took all "prescribed" by me herbs, vitamins, etc. almost religiously.

However, with Harry De Camp report, almost a miracle has happened—my husband read this book almost with enthusiasm!

Frankly speaking, he was really interested in this book.

I saw a hope coming back to him (He was really "down", totally depressed, during his hospital stay, while undergoing the chemotherapy treatment.)

Also, another patient in his room, after reading this book, looked almost like a newly born! He has changed his attitude completely and I saw him "coming back" to life!

After chemotherapy, my husband underwent radiation treatment, during which an area of his abdomen, including the pancreas, was radiated.

I remember that close to the end of this radiation treatment, he started to complain about a severe pain, resembling a burning sensation, in the radiated area of his abdomen. He was very weak and looked pale.

He complained that the radiation treatment was killing him.

I have found a remedy!

I found from the "health books" that the aloe vera juice was helpful in this situation. I bought my husband a bottle of the aloe vera juice, and he was started on this treatment right away.

He hated to drink this juice, its taste—but a "miracle" has happened again!

His pain, the burning sensation, was gone almost in no time after he started to drink this juice! There was no burning sensation in his abdomen any longer! It disappeared!

He felt well again!

Soon after my husband finished the radiation treatment, I put him on a full alternative cancer therapy treatment, which I found as a most beneficial one.

This therapy involved herbs, vitamins, shark cartilage, and special restrictions in his diet.

No, no, he was not a vegetarian—he ate almost "normally" (yes, he even ate "Polish kielbasy"), but in a moderation, and certain foods were totally eliminated from his diet!

He also was seeing his doctor, for a follow-up tests and medical examinations, regularly—doctor F., the surgeon became his "leading" doctor. He always had time to advise my husband about the follow-up tests' results, and to talk to him, while doctor M., the oncologist was always "too busy" to call my husband concerning the tests' results, so we had to wait, anxious and guessing, for the most recent follow-up tests' results.

After some time doctor F. asked my husband, if he were taking any kind of a special "medication" against cancer. He was suspecting, seeing my husband's good health and condition, and a good attitude, that there had to be "something", some "secret" medication, keeping my husband in such good shape!

CHAPTER IX

A LESSON IN MY LIFE

I was alone at my home.

I was thinking about my husband, his health, and our entire situation.

"Even if my husband's cancer comes back,"—I thought,—"What probably wouldn't be the case, not in a nearest future (according to his doctors, this cancer would have reappeared already), even if something "bad" happens to my husband (nobody lives forever), I can say that these three years since my husband was diagnosed and operated for the metastasized pancreatic cancer, were very happy and productive years in his life.

Instead of thinking about the inevitable death sentence, given to him by his doctors, he enjoyed his life. He had been actively working in his profession since operation.

His employer used his knowledge and devotion in work, and he was often asked for a support in solving the most complicated HVAC engineering problems. Also, his employer was sending him all over the United States on business trips.

In his leisure time, he engaged in his favorite activities; in the summer time, he liked camping, swimming in the lakes and ocean, and sailing; and he loved to ski in the wintertime.

The three of us; our eight years old son Raymond; my husband, and I (our older son Michael preferred more his friends' company than ours), we really had great moments together, each summer, at the campsite!

As a handyman, he made all necessary repairs at our home (He was a very talented "gold handyman", and performed not only house but also, car repairs—he had modernized the two old bathrooms in our house; and made a new one, since his operation.)

Instead of thinking about the inevitable death to come, he was very busy with his daily activities which, for sure, included taking all "prescribed" to him by me herbs, and other nutritional supplements, three times daily. I never had to remind him about it!

Though he was still "lazy" with going to church (frankly speaking, I also frequently tried to find some "excuses" as I preferred to pray on my own), I knew that he had found, similarly like I did that God loved all of us, and He also loved him. That God didn't want him to be sick and suffer.

Also, this experience with my husband's sickness enriched my life.

I started to look onto many things in a quite different way than I used to do before.

We still, sometimes, had small disputes (oh, yes, we used to have really big "differences" in the past)—but I looked onto life and its purpose, quite differently.

I understood that life was too short to spend it on arguments and quarrels—and that both sides had to understand it.

I learned that thanks to my experience with my husband's sickness, I was able to understand better the sense of life.

I believe that everybody's life is like a school. We must go through different experiences, like through different lessons, which are taught in school classes, in our life. We have to learn from each of these lessons.

It is a main purpose of our life—to learn. We have to learn, during and from, our life.

We have to learn both from our mistakes and accomplishments.

We have to make mistakes to find out when we were wrong. We have to suffer to find out how to be happy!

We have to learn so we will know how to benefit both from moments of happiness and sadness.

I believe that each of us—you, me, all of us, we get grades from each "lesson" in a life.

Only at the very end of it we will be able to see either if we had successfully passed, or if we failed, our life school.

Do you want to get a good certificate?

Just when I was finishing writing this story, a telephone rung, similarly, like some time

ago. "This is Doctor's F. nurse,"—I heard a voice.

"May I speak to Mr. Ryduchowski, please?"—I felt a pug of anxiety in my chest, again.

"This is Mrs. Ryduchowski speaking. I am his wife, my husband is not at home, do you want to leave a message for him, or maybe, do you prefer to call him at his work?"—I answered.

"I can leave a message for him,"—the lady has advised,—" Please tell your husband that Doctor F.

received and reviewed your husband's most recent follow-up tests. Doctor F. wanted to inform your husband that everything was normal."

"Normal,"—I asked,—"What does it mean?

What about my husband's next visit at the doctor's office?

For when is it scheduled?"

"Which visit?"—she asked.

"I already told you that everything was normal, that there was nothing wrong with your husband's health!

The doctor advised that he didn't need to see him."

"Oh, no,"—I interrupted her—" In my opinion, the doctor should see my husband!

He should see and talk to my husband, and should say him, in person, that my husband was doing great, that the tests didn't show any reappearance of the cancer, that after three years since his operation everything is normal."

Both my husband and I we really appreciated doctor F., his professionalism, and a great, human attitude towards his patients.

"My husband really likes his visits at the doctor's F. office and talking to the doctor, nurse,"—I told the lady.

"Could you please call my husband to tell him what you just told me and ask him if he wants to have an appointment?"—I gave her his office phone number.

As soon as my husband came back home, I smiled and asked him:

"Casimir, did you receive a call from Doctor's F. office?

What did they tell you?"

He looked at me with a stern expression on his face; he tried to sound very serious—"Danusia, doctor F. wants to see me urgently! Maybe, there is something wrong with me?"

I had a long look at my husband—I saw his bold forehead with some remnants of dark hairs turning gray, his funny, mixed-dark -blond mustache, and his gray eyes, full of warmth and wisdom, and now, somehow seriously anxious.

I knew that he was kidding!

And I giggled!

THE END

The cancer came back when we were sure it would never be back.

It took us by a surprise.

In a six weeks time, over four years since his operation and after enjoying a healthy and productive life till its end, my husband was gone. He didn't suffer any pain.

He died in our bedroom. In his last moments, I saw a bizarre expression on his face.

He was looking intensively towards the window, as if he were seeing something or somebody there—and I will never learn what or who it was. Then, he passed away.

Sometimes, I almost believe that he finally passed through the hole in this immense cupola he described to me after his out-of-the-body experience at the St. Barnabas hospital.

His time had come finally. He was not sent back to his sick body at this time. He travelled to another world.

The night after coming back from a hospital where my husband's heart finally stopped to beat, I sat alone in our bedroom.

I looked into the sky—I saw a comet there. It was so close and shinier than most of the stars. It was almost as shiny as a full moon.

www.ingramcontent.com/pod-product-compliance
Lightning Source LLC
Chambersburg PA
CBHW031229280526
45784CB00004B/1502